How to Break a Fast (Appropriately) and Keep the Weight Off

A 30-DAY GUIDE

*Detailed Breaking a Fast Instructions

*Meal Plans for the Long-Term

*Motivation to Press On!

This Book is Volume 6 of The Ongoing Series Entitled: How To Lose Weight Fast, Keep it Off & Renew The Mind, Body & Spirit Through Fasting, Smart Eating & Practical Spirituality

ROBERT DAVE JOHNSTON

Published by:

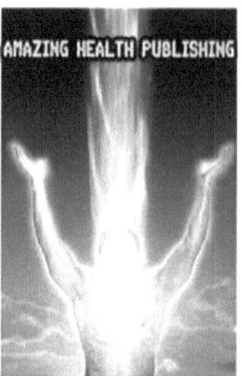

If you are interested in reading new books as they are released, follow Rob on Twitter @FitnessFasting

Copyright

Disclaimer & Legal Notices

The health-related information and suggestions contained in any of the books or written material mentioned above are based on the research, experience and opinions of the Author and other contributors. Nothing herein should be misinterpreted as actual medical advice, such as one would obtain from a Physician, or as advice for self-diagnosis or as any manner of prescription for self-treatment.

Neither is any information herein to be considered a particular or general cure for any ailment, disease or other health issue. The material contained within is offered strictly and solely for the purpose of providing Holistic health education to the general public. Persons with any health condition should consult a medical professional before entering this or any fasting, weight loss, detoxification or health related program.

Even if you suffer from no known illness, we recommend that you seek medical advice before starting any fasting, weight loss and/or detoxification program, and before choosing to follow any advice given this book. For any products or services mentioned or suggested in this book, you should read all packaging and instructions, as no substance, natural or drug, can be guaranteed to work in everyone.

Information and statements regarding dietary supplements, products or services mentioned in this book many not have been evaluated by the Food and Drug Administration and are not intended to diagnose, treat, cure, or prevent any disease. Never disregard or delay in seeking professional medical advice because of something you have read in this book.

Nothing that you read in this book should be regarded as medical or health advice. If you do anything recommended in this book, without the supervision of a licensed medical doctor, you do so at your own risk. Not recommended for persons with any health related condition unless supervised by a qualified health practitioner.

Because there is always some risk involved in any health-related program, the Author, Publisher and contributors assume no responsibility for any adverse effects or consequences resulting from the use of any suggested preparations or procedures described in any of the books or other written materials associated with the website FitnessThroughFasting.com. The author reserves the right to alter and update his opinions based on new conditions at any time.

Dedication

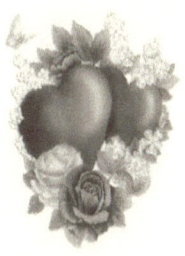

This series of books are dedicated to my mother Sonia Noemi, without whom I would not even be alive today. I love you mom. Thank you for never losing faith in me and supporting me, even when everything seemed hopeless and everyone else had given up on me. I owe you everything. I could collect all of the precious stones on this earth and lay them on your lap, and even still, I would not even come close to giving back to you all that you have given me.

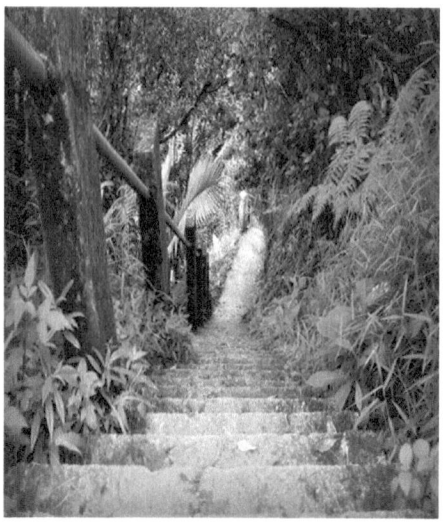

"The 40-day water fast I completed years ago in a Caribbean rainforest was one of the most powerful experiences of my life. BUT, there was one lesson that I still hadn't learned."

Prelude to Disaster

In 1998, I spent 40 days in a men's recovery farm as a volunteer. Located in the mountains of San Juan, Puerto Rico, the farm is near the breathtaking *El Yunque* rainforest. The director of the program, Luis, was around 5 feet, 5 inches tall with curly black hair and tiny eyes that hid behind his thick-rimmed glasses. He also sported a huge potbelly that looked like he was about to give birth to quintuplets. I was going to confront him about his weight when the time was right. Luis was a very gentle man who cared deeply about helping troubled young men straighten out their lives.

And he knew pretty much everything about me: My insane binge eating and drinking episodes, my arrival into the class of *'morbidly obese,'* my destruction of promising writing and music careers, the loss of a wonderful woman who was always willing to stand by me. I loved her, but the binging and drinking turned me into a monster, an animal that lived only on instinct.

"Drink, eat and destroy yourself!" said the

inner demons. "Eat until your belly explodes and end your pathetic little life!" they yelled.

No matter how important the engagement, I'd always opt to lock myself into a motel room with five xtra large pizzas and a case of beer. In isolation, I'd eat and drink until I passed out. I'd wake up (*or come to*) in the morning surrounded by garbage, my body usually drenched with vomit and even urine. Great times, huh? I lost my human dignity and behaved as a rabid dog in search of meat.

Luis knew of my struggles and was always there for me in the early days. After I finished the first 40-day fast, I went down from 296 pounds to 246. I returned to a structured eating plan and, after three months, weighed in at 244. *I had kept the weight off and actually lost two more pounds.* I can't give myself all of the credit, however. I broke the fast with the direct assistance of my mother and grandmother.

They cooked up this vegetable soup that was truly amazing. So those two wonderful ladies are the reason why I didn't go crazy breaking that particular fast. It was all very exciting. After fighting obesity for decades, I had found a discipline that could help me wipe out the blubber and give me a new lease on life. Now I was ready to do another 40-day fast, and this time, with God's help, I would reach my ideal weight of 195-200 pounds. Doing this second fast in the rainforest sounded appealing. There was also a *'fear'* element to it. I'd heard of people who supposedly ran into extraterrestrials while walking through the trails. There are many stories of people who went on walks and never came back; in spite of search parties, they never appeared or were heard from again.

Needless to say, **El Yunque** wields tremendous mystique. Another thing I liked about Luis' home was that there were plenty of animals, including ducks, chickens, cows, bulls, horses and, last but not least, a HUGE 600-pound pig everyone called *The Emperor*. They even drew a nice crown at the top of the sty, the words **The Emperor** written in blue, yellow, green and white. Yes, this was the perfect place. If you walked west, you'd promptly reach the first group of paths that led to the belly of the rainforest. The other men were not allowed to enter the rainforest's trails, but since I was there as a '*volunteer*,' I figured I'd be free to explore to my heart's content, or so I thought. This experience was a huge contrast to my first fast, which I did alone in a room at my grandmother's house. It worked out well, except for the constant offerings of food, people coming in to ask questions and basically interrupting my silence and state of inner observation.

I guess somewhere in the back of my mind I was hoping that something '*unusual*' would happen in this second 40-day water fast, that I could have a spiritual experience of some sort. I was sick of the life that I'd been living; I was hungry for answers... for something better. On the phone, I told Luis that I'd be going up there for 40 days, but, that I'd be fasting, drinking water only. At first he was a bit resistant.

"Oh no, not that fasting again!" he said.

I assured him that I'd be fine, that I needed to do this for physical, mental as well as spiritual reasons. He was present when I finished my first 40-day fast and, in spite of his misgivings, was amazed by the results.

"You look 20 years younger," he told me. "And your skin is glowing... your entire body is glowing! Amazing!"

"Yes," I told him. "Bear in mind that you're next buddy! We got to eliminate that potbelly and return you to optimum health. Your wife and three children deserve a healthy father, don't you think?"

He lowered his head.

"Yes," he whispered. "I just don't think I have that kind of strength."

"Bullcrap!" I retorted angrily. "I've seen you mentor youth who were criminals and hardcore drug addicts. I've seen how your example taught them of a better way. There are dozens of men who are clean and sober today because **YOU** were there to motivate them. So don't tell me that you can't lose the weight. You **CAN**, and you **WILL**!"

So, on that rainy Saturday morning, I packed my clothes in a brown suitcase and tossed it in the back of my 1988 Ford Bronco. I was on my way to the *Hogar de la Santisima Trinidad* (Home of the Holiest Trinity), that's what Luis called the home. As I was pulling out of the garage, my mother and grandmother ran out, seemingly alarmed.

"What's the matter," I said, watching them stand before me with eyes wide open, each one holding white Tupperware bowls filled with a brown, steamy liquid.

"Just in case you can't handle it," said grandma.

"We cooked a very light broth...there's hardly anything in it," my mother added.

"I want you to take it in case you get weak," she continued, "in case you need to eat. It's very light broth."

Initially I felt anger. But I had to smile, seeing their beautiful faces, so worried about me and my insane fasting adventures, worried that I may collapse in the wilderness and not have energy to find my way out. I could certainly understand their concern.

El Yunque National Rainforest is located on the slopes of the *Sierra de Luquillo* Mountains and it encompasses 28,000 acres of land, making it the largest block of public land in Puerto Rico. *El Toro*, the highest mountain peak in the forest rises 1,065 meters (3,494 ft.) above sea level. Ample rainfall (*over 200 inches a year in some* *areas*) creates a jungle-like setting — lush foliage, crags, waterfalls and rivers are a prevalent sight. As you can imagine, there's lots to explore, and there are plenty of opportunities to run into danger, either by getting lost, eating the wrong type of fruit or running into the hoodlums that traipse to and fro at night.

"Why do you always have to do everything in the extreme?" grandma asked, the bowl with broth still in her precious hands. "Why can't you fast for a few days at a time and build from there? But 40 days again! Who do you think you are, Moses?"

"Ha-ha!" I laughed. "No, I'm not Moses. I'm me, and THIS is what I have to do for myself. Please respect that, and keep me in your prayers."

I gave them a hug and a kiss, got on the truck and was off to the rainforest. I made the trip in 2.5 hours. Slowly, I drove the truck up the steep hill, atop of which was the home's entrance; downward slopes on every side of the house led directly into the forest. It was totally surreal, like a place out of time.

A house on top of a hill with a farm in the

surrounding land, a vast rainforest just a few feet away. I remember standing there for several minutes in awe, taking in the spectacular scenery, including a direct view of the "*El Toro*" peak which, northwest from where we stood, rose thousands of feet in the air and touched the very clouds that hovered above the extraordinary mountain range.

"If takes hours to climb to the top of *El Toro*," said one of the guys.

"But once you make it up there, you'll have a 360-degree view of the entire island of Puerto Rico."

"*That is something that I really want to experience,*" I thought.

But my awe and inspiration were promptly quelled. As I walked into the house and greeted some of the guys, Luis came out with a huge grin on his face.

"Here's your cook," he told the men.

"What!" I shrieked. "This is a sick joke, right?"

"Nope. For the next 40 days, you're the cook," Luis repeated.

Half smiling and grimacing, I pulled him into the adjacent laundry room. The sound of washers and dryers was perfect to drown the anger I was about to dump on this gentleman.

"What the hell is your problem Luis? You know that I'm going to be fasting. Why would you make me the cook?"

Luis looked into my eyes and smiled.

"Maybe God wants to know just how committed you are," he replied. "Fasting in isolation is one thing, but fasting while cooking meals three times a day, now that's some real discipline, self-restraint and commitment."

I was in real trouble. This wasn't going to be a vacation with some easy tasks here and there as I had hoped. I'd have to cook three meals every day for FIFTY men! *"How the heck am I supposed to pull that off?"* I thought.

Well, I don't want to bore you with details. Let it be said that it was one of the hardest experiences of my life. Handling chicken, fish, steak, rice, beans and even dessert pushed me to the very edge of my human strength. With me, the fasting hunger pangs usually go away (*at least a little*) by days 11 to 14.

Here, however, the hunger never went away.

My stomach hurt and, to make matters worse, I was having a hard time sleeping. When fasting, sleeping for me is a wonderful oasis where I can hide, for a little while. But, for some reason or another, I slept only in one-hour spurts. I'd wake up exhausted, hungry and in a terrible mood.

That morning, trying to pick up a garbage bin, I pulled my lower back. I was fine for the rest of the day, but by the next morning I was in excruciating pain and could hardly walk. To get around, I used a thick piece of wood I found around the farm. Now I really looked like Moses!

I was hungry and responsible to cook for 50 men, but now I also was in a great deal of pain.

Luis would bring in bags of ice so that I could lie on them; that helped a lot. The swelling, however, continued to get worse. This happened at around day 34. I had shown up weighing 245 pounds and was now at 205! I was within ten pounds of my goal! The last ten days were the biggest test of all. I was hungry, tired, angry, sporting a thick beard and in constant pain... definitely not in the greatest of moods. Luis saw my condition.

"Here is where most men take their hands off the plow," he said. "Why don't you come inside and have a nice meal and lay on ice for a few hours. You'll feel a lot better."

I looked at him silently for a few moments, then I smiled.

"That's the first mistake you've made with me Luis. If you tell me to quit, I'm going to do the opposite. I'm bullheaded and intractable, remember?"

Luis let out a huge belly laugh.

"I was counting on that!" he said.

For the last ten days I learned a lot about suppressing hunger, pain and mood swings so that I could be there for others. When I put aside my own complaints, I realized that many of these men were in terrible situations. Some were homeless, some had HIV, some were on their way to prison, some had lost their wives and children, and some didn't care and were going back to their addictions. And here I was complaining about my little hunger, lack of sleep and back pain! My attitude totally changed in those days. Normally, if I was in a bad mood, I'd disappear and not talk to anybody. Here, since I was the cook, I was always amidst the guys and got to hear about their lives and trials. In whatever feeble way I could, I tried to help. I decided to ignore my human wants and desires and place myself in the hands of the *Creator*, to do with me as **He** wished. I kept a thorough journal where I placed my inmost thoughts and feelings. I still read it today, and I cherish the amazing nuggets that I wrote there. One part in particular impacted me tremendously. In it, I wrote:

"You are already complete in every way and are lacking absolutely nothing. Let your peace and joy be full by realizing that, in all ways, you are whole and complete. The Father shows you all things, takes you to all things and brings you all things. You need and are lacking nothing. Let your joy be complete."

By the time day 40 arrived, I weighed 196

pounds, a solid loss of 40 pounds. I had never seen myself this thin. I couldn't stop going to the mirror to look at myself. I yelled in victory. I wept. One of the skinnier guys in the home gave me a pair of his jeans, waist size 33. And they fit me perfectly! I couldn't wait to get my hands on my old 46 waist size pants and toss them in the trash. Size 33, me? Now I could finally go to the beach and take off my shirt! Wow! I felt great satisfaction. **BUT**, there was a very important lesson that I had **NOT** learned.

Sure, I saw how I could set aside my own wants and pains and, instead, focus on the needs of another. I saw how I could suppress my own hunger and still cook for 50 men three times a day. And many other things I learned during that fast. **BUT**, sadly, I had no clue how to properly break a fast to ensure long-term weight loss and health. My happiness for being thin would be short-lived.

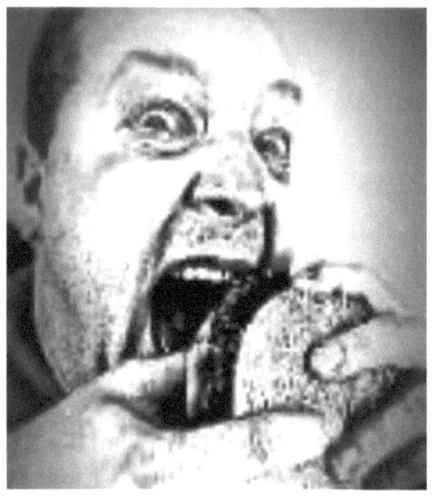

"Coming off a victorious 40-day water fast, feeling slim and on a spiritual high, I told Luis I was ready to break the fast with the group. Tonight's menu: Cheeseburgers."

The Cheeseburger Fiasco

Having reached my weight objective, I told Luis that the fasting was over and that now it was time to celebrate. Still hurting from the back injury, I asked some of the guys if they could lite the barbecue and cook up some meat patties for cheeseburgers. I recall feeling that I probably wasn't being too smart.

That I should break the fast with something lighter, like juice or soup.

But I waved the thoughts off, rationalizing that, after all of the pain and discomfort I just went through, <u>I deserved to enjoy</u>. I came out of my cabin a half hour later to find dozens of cheeseburgers laying on top of the picnic table where the men usually ate. Without thinking, I grabbed one and pretty much inhaled it in less than thirty seconds. I grabbed another and did the same. In less than 15 minutes, I ate three or four cheeseburgers, all along slapping myself in the back for a *'job well done.'*

Then everything fell apart.

Ten or fifteen minutes later I began to have stabbing pains in the center of my stomach.

It literally felt as though somebody was sticking a knife into my gut. As the minutes passed, the pain got worse and worse. I ran to the bathroom in hopes of moving the bowels.

When I entered the bathroom and turned on the light, I came face to face with myself in the mirror.

To my horror, my eyes were surrounded by dark circles, almost black. It looked as though somebody had painted them with a marker. Nausea hit me and I vomited for a few minutes. But the stomach pain kept increasing. Then, when I looked down at my belly, I saw that it was inflated like a balloon. At this point I totally panicked and asked Luis to please take me to a hospital.

"Why?" he asked. "What's the matter?"

"I made a huge mistake," I replied. "I broke the fast badly and I think I'm in great danger... I think I may be dying."

Within 35 minutes we pulled into a nearby hospital. By then, my belly had continued to swell; it looked like it was about to burst. The black circles around my eyes were expanding outwards towards the cheeks.

The stomach pain was excruciating. When we walked into the hospital, I was literally yelling out loud from the pain. I could hardly keep myself upward. Soon after, I collapsed. All I remember are nurses running over with a stretcher and taking me into one of the exam rooms. I kept shouting and squirming in the stretcher; it felt like my intestines were going to burst. Not able to really speak, it fell on Luis to explain to the doctor what had happened.

"He did what?" the doctor said. "Are you crazy?" he said, looking at me.

"Yes!" I yelled in agony. "I'm crazy... definitely crazy, thanks for pointing that out doc!"

It was promptly decided that they would pump my stomach to remove as much of the food as possible. Then I would have to go through a series of enemas to help empty the digestive system. I developed a high fever and couldn't stop shivering. I continued to vomit every ten to fifteen minutes. I'd get the urge to move my bowels, but when I sat in the toilet, the pain back there was excruciating, as if I was trying to pass a volleyball. The nurses also gave me a variety of stool softeners in hopes that I would soon be able to pass those cursed cheeseburgers.

All told, I spent three days in the hospital, two of them in intensive care because my stomach lining almost ruptured. If that had happened, I would have died a very painful and horrible death. After I left the hospital, I continued to feel sick for at least two weeks. I was stricken with chronic diarrhea and intermittent abdominal pain. All I could eat were soups and fruit juices. Finally, nearly 30 days after I broke the fast with cheeseburgers, the symptoms subsided and I was healthy again. What is the moral of this story?

That breaking a fast is a delicate process.

If you don't do it properly, at the very least you will gain all of the weight back and have to do it all over again. At the very worst, breaking a fast inappropriately could lead to serious illness and possibly death. I hope that my gross (*and extremely embarrassing*) mistake will help you to understand that what we're doing here is very serious business. I certainly got the message. I have spent years researching the topic of properly breaking a fast. While there are many methods out there, the one that I will share with you here is the one that I've found most effective. Now that I've totally made a jackass out of myself with this story, let's move forward with our 30-day program!

PS: About five years later, Luis called me and said he had begun a juice fast. He hung on for 90 days and lost 110 pounds. From what I've heard, he's kept the weight off and now even runs marathons in San Juan as well as in the US mainland. God bless him; he is truly a remarkable man.

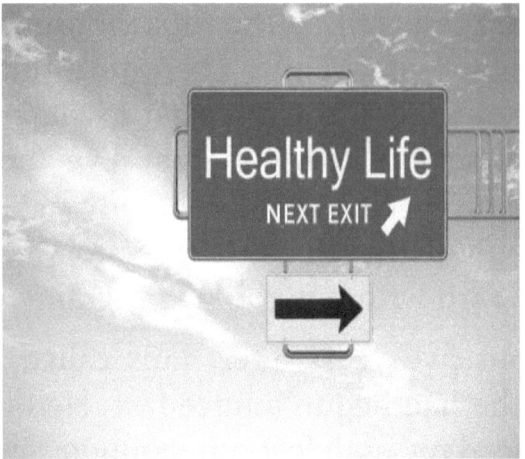

"Do not let anything sway you away from your vision; not hunger, not mood swings, not friends, family, not **ANYONE**! This is <u>YOUR</u> moment to shine and achieve all of your weight loss and health-improvement goals!"

A Clear Vision

By far, the **NUMBER ONE** question that I receive from Fitness Through Fasting.com visitors is:

How Do I Keep The Weight Off After Fasting?

I literally get dozens of such emails on an ongoing basis, many of them from good people that have lost huge amounts of weight with fasting and/or dieting. However, within a few months they have gained it all back. There are many who are long-time *fasters and dieters*, yet they still are unable to keep the weight off once they start the *re-feeding* process (*re-feeding is what I call the process of starting to eat after a period of fasting or strict dieting*) Why is it so hard to keep the weight off? And what can be done to solve this problem? Well, that is what this book is all about.

Before I start, however, I'd like to make a clarification: during the first month of breaking a fast, **EVERYONE** will usually gain back a few pounds. The specific numbers will vary depending on how much weight was lost. If a person lost, say 60 pounds during a 40-day water fast, it is common to see a gain of 5 to 10 pounds in the first two weeks of re-feeding. Please do not be alarmed. There is good reason for this initial weight gain. The metabolism slows down while fasting. That means that the body will consume energy at a slower rate than it does when you're eating. This is often referred to as *starvation mode.* Starvation mode is the body's way of *conserving* resources amidst what it perceives to be a threat to its survival (*fasting*).

Therefore, when you start re-feeding, the metabolism will, initially, run very slowly; it will hoard what you eat and drink in order to create a <u>reserve</u> that will help it get through another crisis. In addition, while hunger normally goes away after 9-11 days of fasting, it comes back with a vengeance once you start re-feeding. Put all of these factors together and we have a pretty good explanation as to why it is so easy to gain weight after fasting or dieting.

But do not despair. If you break the fast appropriately and then adopt healthy eating habits, the body will eventually "*lower its guard*" and reshape itself at the reduced weight you achieved through fasting or dieting. The strategy that I share with you in this book represents a foundation of permanent weight loss. If you are thorough in following the instructions, you **NEVER** have to regain the weight ... ever! The problem is that many people see the inevitable 5-to-10-pound weight-gain and rapidly become discouraged. They get struck by the "*screw it*" syndrome. In many cases, that means giving up and succumbing to old (*and destructive*) eating habits. And when one has been battling binging and compulsive overeating for years, relapsing can happen very quickly. One man wrote me:

"Robert, I don't know what happened. I was doing great for ten days and then, out of nowhere, I ordered a pepperoni pizza. What is the matter with me?"

Nothing is the matter with him. Bad habits do not die without a fight. After fasting, **THAT** is when the real challenge begins. If you think that because you fasted for 40 days "*you are done,*" then you are leaving yourself open for disaster, just like it happened to me after the rainforest fast. The healthy life that you want is at your fingertips, but you will have to prepare yourself for resistance - particularly during the first 9-months-to-a-year of re-feeding. As the history of mankind has shown us: **FREEDOM CARRIES SACRIFICE**. Self-mastery is no different. If you want this to be easy and require no discomfort, then you will likely have a very hard time attaining your goals.

<u>**BUT PLEASE**</u>: be encouraged! There **IS** a way out. It may be tough at first (*there is no magic pill*), but it gets easier over time. In the measure that you stick to your guns, you will grow in character and emotional maturity which, in turn, will give you further insulation against the "*sick*" part of the mind that wants to take you back to unhealthy eating. I want you to go into this with a clear vision of your objective. Do not let anything sway you away from that vision; not hunger, not mood swings, not friends, family, not **ANYONE**! This is <u>YOUR</u> moment to shine and achieve all of your weight loss and health-improvement goals!

How to Use This Book

Please make sure to read this book <u>in its entirety</u> several times before you actually start following the instructions. Make absolutely certain that you have made all the needed preparations. Start fasting with the assurance that you know and understand the instructions! Since I have no idea how long you intend to fast, I'm going to provide detailed instructions for breaking a prolonged one. In other words, a fast lasting longer than fourteen days. If you fasted for shorter than that, don't worry. You **still** can use the same directions. Therefore, I will show you how to break a fast over a period of TEN days. I have found that to be the best timeframe. Then, for the subsequent TWENTY days, I'll give you a very specific (*and simple*) diet to follow. This will be PHASE II of breaking the fast. Altogether, in this book **you will have detailed re-feeding instructions for 30 days.** That gives you a full month of structured, clean and very effective re-feeding. To conclude, I will give you some basic ground rules to follow as you move to PHASE III - **beyond day 30**.

VERY IMPORTANT: If you want this to work, then follow **ALL** of the instructions that I have outlined for you. I am always mystified by some people who ask me for help and support *"while fasting,"* but then brush me aside when it's time to start re-feeding. Many of them write me some time later to say that they gained the weight back and are heartbroken. If you want me to help you, then **LET ME HELP YOU!** **DO NOT** skip steps or try to figure it out on your own. That is why you have me... take the thinking out of the equation and simply take the action. That is what produces **REAL** results. Ok, enough blabbing. Let's get to the meat! (*no pun intended*)

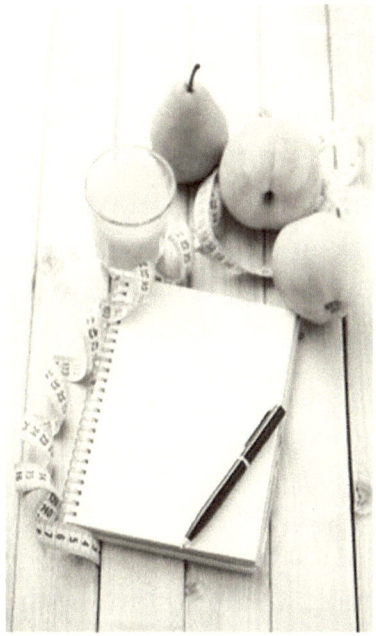

"The stricter you are with the process of breaking a fast, the greater the benefits and the stronger your foundation will be for long-term success. And long-term success is what we want, right?"

Breaking the Fast

Breaking a fast is the most important part of the fasting process. I have run into many people who fast for thirty days and more... but they break it inappropriately. This is unwise and dangerous. The digestive system has been inactive.

We have to wake it up slowly and steadily.

You can literally place your life in danger if you do not break a fast adequately. Just look at what happened to me. Here I am, coming off a great fast in the mountains, and I mess everything up by eating cheeseburgers! I was well intentioned... but not properly informed. So we must tread carefully. Not only that, but I want you to come face-to-face with hunger and **NOT** give in to it. Hunger comes back strong when one breaks a fast.

The key is to stick to the schedule I have outlined.

Do not "*hurry*" things because you "*think*" that you are ready. I have fallen prey to that mental trickery and can tell you that it is **NO FUN**. It takes hard work to complete a fast.

There is nothing more discouraging than to give away the benefits at the last moment with a binge. That is like the man whose boat sinks in the deep sea and he is forced to swim for days in the cold, dark ocean. Finally, he sees the beach up ahead but, just as he is about to touch land, he decides to give up and stop swimming. So, he sinks to the bottom like a piece of lead and drowns. What! All of that swimming for nothing? No way! **Here's my point**: The stricter you are with the process of breaking a fast, the greater the benefits and the stronger your foundation will be for long-term success. And **LONG TERM** success is what we want, right? Right!

Supplies You Will Need

First and foremost you are going to need a juicer. Most people already have one. If you do not, you can usually find them at your local discount store for as little as $20. If you can afford it, I'd suggest that you get a good and sturdy one. All you have to do is search for 'juicers' in Amazon.com and you'll get pages and pages of excellent and affordable models. Please do not disregard this requirement and break the fast with just any juice. I want you to roll up your sleeves and prepare it from whole fruits and veggies.

That's where the real power is!

Once you have the hardware, then it's time to get the produce. During the last few days of your fast, go to the market and pick up some supplies.

Here's my personal "breaking a fast" fruit/veggie combination:

Apples, Pears, Oranges, Celery, Carrots, Spinach, Cucumbers and, last but not least, the mighty watercress.

Your body will receive a tremendous jolt of nutrition. Of course if you have a personal juicing recipe, go ahead and use it. But make sure that you combine <u>**BOTH**</u> fruits and vegetables. Set aside at least two apples and two pears for **eating only**. Don't juice them. We will need them as part of the re-feeding process. Also from the produce section, get some lettuce, tomatoes and a couple of lemons.

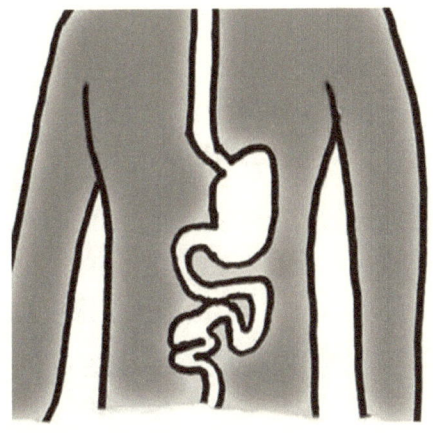

In addition to the produce, you'll need a bottle of <u>Probiotics</u> to help **repopulate the "good bacteria" in your stomach**. Check in the dairy section to see if you find <u>Kefir</u>. Unlike yogurt which contains transient bacteria that do not repopulate the digestive tract, Kefir has active, growing and *"living bacteria"*. This is a marvelous boost to your system, and will swiftly repopulate the digestive tract.

Moreover, get some chicken broth packets, some low-fat milk, a bag of <u>flax seeds</u>, a small bottle of olive oil and a package of some good <u>oat bran cereal</u> (*not the sugar-filled commercial type please!*). These items can usually be found at the health-food section of many supermarkets. If not, then you can order them online. I have added some Amazon.com links above for your convenience. Amazon, in my experience, is cheap and fast.

Finally, purchase a bottle of some natural juice. I use grape and orange, but you can choose whatever type you like best, even vegetable juice. **Keep it simple**. A good juice from the health-food section in your local supermarket will more than suffice.

After day three you will be juicing a combination of fruit and vegetable juice. But for starters, a good bottled **NATURAL JUICE** is enough. That is the end of the shopping list! Please make sure to have all of these items in place prior to the last day of your fast. Do not wait until the last moment. Now let's look at your daily re-feeding schedule. When you are ready to break the fast, start with the following chapter.

Re-Feeding: Day 1

Upon arising, drink two large glasses of water. Over the next hour, meditate on all that has transpired over the course of your fast. If you were keeping a journal (*I strongly recommend it*), take some final notes. Talk about how you are feeling mentally, physically, emotionally etc...

If you practice a specific religion, pray and "*turn over*" the fast to the God of your understanding. You have done A LOT of work. You have shown courage, steadfastness and faith. Once you feel satisfied with your prayer/meditation/journaling time, break the fast with an eight-to-twelve-ounce glass of watered-down juice.

NOTE: This is a very powerful moment. Do not drink the juice nonchalantly. What you have done has great significance for you, your future and for your loved ones. Make sure you drink the juice sitting down and with a thankful and prayerful heart. Some people like to gather their immediate family and have a small celebration.

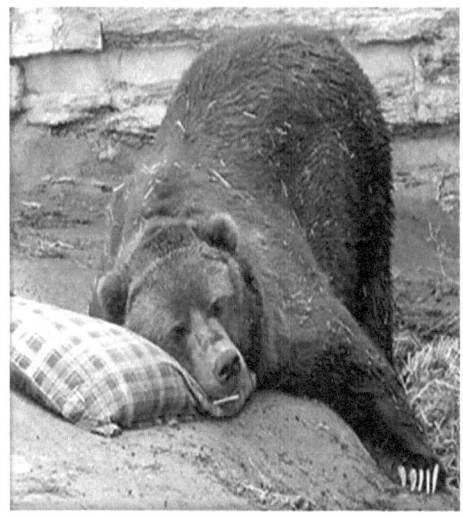

Drink the watered-down juice. One glass only please! Remember: the digestive system has been dormant (*like the sleeping bear above!*) and needs to be roused VERY SLOWLY. You don't want to make the bear angry, do you?

Wait TWO hours and drink another glass of watered-down juice. Drink two more glasses of water. You should feel no irritation or discomfort. If you do, then you will need to dilute the juice even more. To keep it safe, I suggest you mix it 50-50. **Continue to drink a glass every three-to-four hours for the rest of the day**. Make sure to consume at the very least half a gallon of water throughout the day. Keep a fasting journal close and write any thoughts and feelings you may have. The first few days of breaking a fast are filled with deep introspection and insight. Make sure to take the personal time to do just that. Good job! This brings to conclusion your first day of breaking the fast.

Re-Feeding Day 2

Upon arising, immediately drink two large glasses of water (*I recommend you adopt this as a lifetime practice*). Again spend some time in your journal writing your thoughts, ideas and feelings. Write about how you are feeling physically.

You may start to sense greater hunger at this point. It is important to remain vigilant. The mind may attempt to "*convince you*" that you are fine and can go straight to solid food. Don't do it! We want to lay the strongest foundation possible, remember?

For breakfast, drink an eight-to-twelve-ounce glass of your watered-down juice. Today, however, you can reduce the water content by 25%. Stir it well. Drink it slowly. Drink another glass in three-to-four hours.

If, three hours later, you feel ZERO discomfort or irritation, you can start to drink the juice without watering it down. Again, you should not feel any abdominal pain or irritation. If so, then return to the 50-50 dilution for another twelve hours. I can give you detailed instructions, but it is crucial that you listen to your own body and use common sense accordingly.

Better to dilute the juice for another half day than to take any risk. **Please, please listen to your body and proceed with much caution**. If all goes well, you will have finished the day drinking pure juice. Your digestive system will definitely start to reawaken. Ok! This brings to conclusion your second day of breaking a fast.

Re-Feeding: Day 3

Upon arising, drink two large glasses of water. For breakfast drink a glass of your juice, and then take some time to prepare the juicing mix. Go to the Juice Fasting page if need a refresher on juicing. The instructions there are very comprehensive. Prepare one gallon of juice, usually sufficient for three days. Make sure to add at least two tablespoons of pulp into the jug after you're done juicing. **IF** you find that you did not get enough produce to yield a full gallon, add a cup or two of water.

By mid-to-late afternoon you should have finished preparing the juice.

Fill up an eight-to-twelve-ounce glass and sit down in the kitchen table, or wherever you are. This juice will take you to the next level because it contains much more sustenance, fiber, pulp and nutrients than the juice you drank the first two days.

Take a break of at least 10-to-15 minutes and enjoy the juice. It will taste like heaven, trust me. *Drink it slowly and savor the pulp as it hits your tongue*. Chew and savor it as this powerhouse of nutrients goes down your throat to your eagerly-awaiting belly.

What a glorious moment! You completed your fast, and now you are celebrating by breaking it slowly and honoring your body for all of the cleansing, weight loss and healing that it has done.

Thank your body for its loyalty, even at times when you mistreated it.

Make a covenant with yourself that <u>NO MORE</u>.... from this day forward you will eat and live healthy... even if that means going against what others are doing. *You are on the road less traveled*. You are on the road to a much better and vibrant life. If so moved, take out your journal and write whatever comes to your mind.

Spend some time in contemplation, listening to that internal Voice... that gentle, small Voice in your belly that wants to give you direction, revelation, knowledge and deep insight. Pay attention! This Voice is speaking.... even now as you read this! Make sure to refrigerate and cover the juice so that no light enters because it can spoil it prematurely.

In another three-to-four hours you can drink another glass of the juice. At night, make sure not to drink after 10pm. If you are awake and hungry, drink two large glasses of water or crack open a seltzer. A cup of soothing chamomile tea will also help. Remember, as the digestive system reawakens, so does the hunger monster.

You have to be extremely careful and vigilant.

If you are new to fasting, then you may not have been eating all that great. As I said at the beginning, old habits, behaviors and belief systems will attempt to regain control of your life. They will try to enslave you once more. Do **NOT** allow it! Stay alert and focused!

Yes, the fast is over. But this is not the time to lower your guard. Food cravings are cunning and will always look for ways to make you fall. If you can accept that reality, then your chances for long-term success will be much greater. Congratulations! That concludes your third day of breaking a fast.

Re-Feeding: Day 4

Upon arising, immediately drink two large glasses of water. Some people have a watery bowel movement the morning of the fourth post-fasting day. If you do, then that is a clear sign that the digestive system has resumed its duties. But don't worry if you don't; more than likely it won't happen for another day or two.

At your usual breakfast time, go to the refrigerator and take out the jug of juice you prepared yesterday. Shake it vigorously so that the pulp mixes in well. Making sure that the lid is safely in place, turn the jug upside down and shake it some more.

Pour yourself a glass and sit down to drink. Look at the contents and observe the colors and small particles of pulp floating around. You are looking at pure nutrition and health, amazing huh? Continue to take this morning time to write in your journal, recording how you are feeling physically and mentally. If you have any spiritual readings that you are accustomed to doing, then by all means do so.

For the rest of the day, drink a glass of juice every three-to four hours, not exceeding 64 ounces or "8" eight-ounce glasses. No juice should be drunk after 10pm at night. In the measure that you drink the juice, pour water into the jug to replenish. We don't want to water it down too much. However, if you are careful, adding some water will "*stretch*" the yield for up to four and even five days. Another good way to extend the yield is to add some veggie juice into the jug.

Some people ask me if it is okay to add ice to the juice. The answer is YES, but do it sparingly. Do <u>NOT</u> turn the juice into a frozen beverage please! You should not feel any discomfort or irritation. For hunger, increase your water consumption and rely on seltzer and tea. You are doing a great job. Make sure to get plenty of sleep and do not overexert yourself physically.

The body is getting stronger, but it still needs some time. This concludes day four of breaking a fast.

Re-Feeding: Day 5

Upon arising, immediately drink two large glasses of water. You may or may not have a bowel movement at this point. Today we are ready to move to yet another phase of breaking the fast. At your usual breakfast time, go to the refrigerator and take out **ONE** apple and **ONE** pear.

Cut the fruit into four slices each, pour yourself a glass of water and sit down to eat. One apple and one pear is more than enough initially. Chew slowly and wash the fruit down with lots of water. This is your first real "*solid*" food, so it will taste like the nectar of the gods! Enjoy it... you worked hard and deserve it!

Wait **EIGHT** hours. Sit down and eat another plate of fruit as you did earlier. Today you can drink juice every **TWO** hours. So utilize it to hold you up during the day when hunger strikes.

Make sure to continue to drink at least half a gallon of water daily throughout the process.

The digestive system will thank you for it! If you are accustomed to going to the gym or taking part in some type of physical activity, today you can resume, albeit at a reduced capacity.

You will likely find yourself struggling with hunger. Just drink lots of water and seltzer. **DO NOT** give in to the desire to eat more than what is allowed. I want you to receive **maximum benefit from your efforts**. Breaking the fast slowly and steadily is very effective. Do not eat or drink any more juice after 10pm. That is more than enough for today. Goodnight!

Re-Feeding: Day 6

Upon arising, immediately drink two large glasses of water. In the majority of cases, you will have a bowel movement at some point today. If not, you certainly will by tomorrow. For breakfast, take out an apple or pear (*whatever you like most*) and cut it into small pieces.

Go to the cupboard and grab the oat bran cereal you purchased. Measure out **ONE** cup and pour it into a bowl. Add **ONE** cup of low-fat milk. Sprinkle the fruit on top. Sit down to eat! This is yet another phase.

Now we are giving the digestive system some oats and bran... which will help immensely. Again, the hunger will want you to inhale the cereal. **Don't!** Eat slowly, taking care to chew the food up to 30 times before swallowing. When you are done eating, take one *Probiotics* capsule.

How are you feeling? This is the most you have eaten since you broke the fast! Is the food going down smooth? Any pains, aches in the belly? You should not have any. If you do, then go back one day and eat fruit only for another 24 hours. If all is well, you can eat one apple and one pear in eight hours and drink a glass of juice every two hours - just like yesterday. By the end of the day, the juice should pretty much be gone. Great job!

At dinnertime (*no later than 8pm*), take out the lettuce, cucumbers and tomatoes and make yourself a salad. We don't want this salad to be **HUGE**, so don't eat with your eyes. *Half a head of lettuce, a cucumber and a tomato will more than suffice.* For dressing, add a tiny amount of olive oil and a squeeze of lemon. Mix it well. Sit down to eat with a large glass of water. Again, eat slowly and **chew each bite until it dissolves in your mouth**. Take your time and enjoy. Drink a full glass of water when done.

Great job! If you get hungry for the rest of the night, drink more water and/or seltzer. How about a cup of soothing chamomile tea? Allow at least two hours after eating before you go to bed. If you can go for a short walk, that would be terrific.

Have a good night!

Re-Feeding: Day 7

Upon arising, immediately drink two large glasses of water. Today is going to be **EXACTLY** like yesterday, including the Probiotics in the morning after your cereal. At around 2 or 3pm, however, mix a heaping tablespoon of flax seed into an eight or twelve ounce glass of water or juice. Drink it! Eat your salad at night and make sure to continue to drink lots of water.

For certain, your bowels will be moving. When you go, it should be easy and effortless... no straining. Those are the amazing benefits of a super clean digestive system! Excellent. That's it for today.

Re-Feeding: Day 8

Upon arising, drink two glasses of water. Today will be exactly like yesterday. Cereal, fruit and low-fat milk in the morning with your Probiotics and flax seed mixed with water or juice in the afternoon.

At night, however, make yourself a cup of chicken broth. INSTEAD of the usual salad, today you can also have steamed vegetables in small quantities. (*I like broccoli, carrots, squash and cauliflower*). You are allowed small sprinkles of olive oil, salt and parmesan cheese for either the salad or veggies.

The broth and veggies are the largest meal to date! Eat slowly and chew well. DO NOT gorge! Seriously, I have known people who break long fasts with huge plates of vegetables marinated with olive oil and salt. That's sheer insanity. It's not just about what you are eating; it also has a lot to do with quantity.

When breaking a fast, it is best NOT to bombard the system with large amounts of food – even if it is vegetables. Eat, but take it easy. Again, you MUST resist the desire to overeat. If you get careless, you will pay for it with physical and emotional discomfort. So **PLEASE** (*pretty please!*) be careful. That concludes day eight of breaking an extended water fast.

Re-Feeding: Day 9

Upon arising, immediately drink two large glasses of water. Today will be exactly like yesterday. Oat bran cereal in the morning with sliced fruit and low-fat milk. Probiotics. More fruit during the day accompanies by flax seed beverage in the afternoon, and your broth and salad (*or veggies*) at night.

Re-Feeding: Day 10

On the TENTH day after the fast, start with your usual glasses of water, oat bran cereal and fruit. Now it's time to go to the market and stock up for the **Phase II STANDARD DIET.** Yes, that means that you finally get to eat a little more.

But if you followed the last nine days as I instructed, you have protected your fasting efforts like a lioness would her little cubs. This is what has to be done. Slow is fast, remember? Yes, if you take each step slowly and with a clear structure, the risk of relapse is notably lessened. And, after all, that is what we want, correct?

A note of warning: *Here is where many people fall off the wagon and start to backslid with their diet. The hunger will be notable since, even though you broke the fast, you still are eating substantially less than you normally would. So the physical hunger is normal, and so are mood swings and irritability.*

Have you ever seen how mad Fred Flintstone would get when he was hungry? Yes, you might even growl. So what? Growl away... but **DO NOT** give in! This is a very important transition. To do it properly it must be carried out with great caution, and follow the specific menu that I'm about to give you... ok?

While I use countless diet combinations, below is one that helped me to break 25 years of obesity and binge eating. I completed a 40-day water fast, did the ten-day re-feeding EXACTLY as described above, and then switched to this. So I am going to make it ultra-easy for you by simply telling you what do to and expecting it to be carried out exactly as instructed. I told you I would give you direct instructions, and that is what we are going to do here. Right now, let's look at the simple diet you will follow during the next 20 days.

Standard Diet

Starting today, and for the next 20 days, follow this diet:

Breakfast 8:00 AM

Plain Oatmeal – NOT INSTANT! - prepared with skim milk ONLY. Replace sugar by adding dates, prunes and/or raisins into the oatmeal. You can interchange the oatmeal with the *"lowest sugar"* breakfast cereal you can find. I personally use Total and All Bran. After the meal drink a large glass of water. Eat NOTHING else.

*4-6 egg whites mixed with the vegetables of your choice for a veggie omelet

*One cup of decaffeinated coffee with a sprinkle of skim milk

I strongly suggest that you stay away from artificial sweeteners. I've been using **Stevia** for some time now. At first I didn't like it because it tends to be slightly bitter. But I've gotten used to it and do not use anything else. This is important because, for most of us, sugar was always an issue. Training yourself to cut down (*or eliminate*) sugar intake is one of the most powerful things you can do for your health and weight.

Lunch - Noon

Three corn tortillas (*no bread, even if it is whole grain! You can find corn tortillas at the bread aisle in your local supermarket*) with lean turkey or tuna (*no mayo!*), lettuce and tomato – and a very light sprinkle of olive oil and salt (*sea salt is best*). Drink a large glass of water before and after the meal. Eat Nothing Else!

Snack: 3-4PM

A cup of dates, prunes and/or raisins mixed with non-fat yogurt as dessert. OR,

One Apple, 5 sticks of celery and 6 sticks of baby carrots. Glass of water.

Dinner 7-8PM

As many as three steamed skinless chicken breasts or fish fillets (*preferably wild fish*). Steamed vegetables of your choice (*I recommend broccoli & cauliflower*) and a healthy side salad with: lettuce, tomato, cucumbers, alfalfa and a light sprinkle of olive oil and salt. Drink a large glass of water before and after the meal.

Nighttime Snack 10PM

One apple or pear. A cup of chamomile tea. Chamomile tea is very soothing to the stomach and will relax you so that you can rest.

Please do <u>NOT</u> eat anything else after 10PM. You will, in essence, **be fasting every night from 10PM until breakfast time the following day.** This daily fast is an important part of the process because it will teach your stomach to go for extended hours without food. At first you might find yourself very hungry in the middle of the night. Simply drink two large glasses of water and go back to bed. In time, the hunger will go away, and you will wake up feeling like a million bucks! If you have trouble sleeping, take one or two 500 mg tabs of <u>Tryptophan</u>. I use it all the time and it works great.

That's it! The diet is very simple and easy to put together. It brings eating back to basics. In essence, it forces the stomach to get used to smaller quantities of food, which is required for the long-term weight loss that you want.

Additional Tips

You can make the dinner salad as large as you want it, but the rest of the meals are to be followed exactly as written.

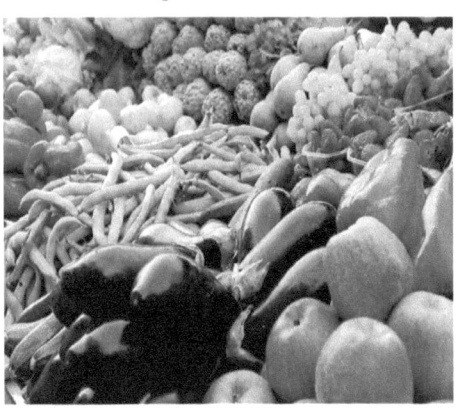

For Vegans:

If you are a vegetarian, you can replace the poultry and fish for plant-sourced protein in small quantities. The best choice is simple well-cooked whole grain and bean combinations. The smaller the bean, the easier it is to digest. Mung beans are well-known for their cleansing and protective attributes.

Whole mung beans can be sprouted and eaten like a vegetable. **Brown rice and red lentils are another good complete protein combination**. Nuts and seeds also provide protein but are high in fat and best eaten fresh in very small quantities or avoided altogether. Making these variations, you will have no trouble following this diet – even if you are a total vegan as many of my colleagues are.

Seasoning the Fish and/or Chicken

Make sure the fish or chicken pieces have been thoroughly washed. Squeeze fresh lemon on both sides of the meat. Look for a non-salt seasoning of garlic powder & herbs at your local supermarket. There are many non-salt seasonings. The one mentioned above is just a suggestion.

Add the seasoning according to your taste. Then add some salt (*sea salt if possible*) to taste. It is better to add the salt separately and be able to control the amounts. Most conventional seasonings are way too high on salt and should be avoided. You can then add a sprinkle of extra virgin olive oil. Use the oil very sparingly. A final option is to add a very light touch of apple cider vinegar for additional taste.

To Cook

Sprinkle the pan with a light coat of canola Spam spray and some extra virgin olive oil.

Turn the stove to medium heat. Place the fish and or chicken on the pan. Allow it to brown on both sides with the pan "partially covered."

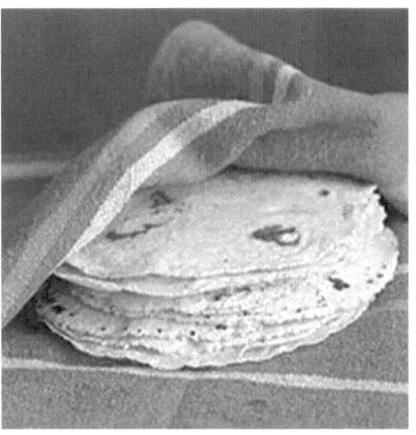

Corn Tortillas

I have found corn tortillas to be an excellent low-calorie substitution to bread and I highly recommend you use them as instructed. But it is important to toast them; otherwise they taste raw and bland. You can heat them in a pan with a very light sprinkle or no-fat spread and allow them to brown on both sides. Or, you can microwave them for about two minutes to get them crunchy.

Once I got used to eating them, I found myself eating tortillas all the time in place of bread. In addition to drinking regular water throughout the day, I recommend seltzer with a squeeze of lemon or lime as it will help settle your tummy and reduce hunger pangs. No sodas of any kind are to be drunk, even if they are "*diet*".

During the day, a hot cup of <u>Green Tea</u> can do wonders to reduce hunger and give you a pep of energy. You can visit the link and read an entire page about green tea and how it can help. I know this all looks like a very tall order. Honestly, IT IS - especially if you are new to this way of eating. But we are not going to take any shortcuts. It is crucial that you follow this plan and continue to give the metabolism the time it needs to speed up and get used to healthy eating.

About Caffeine & Nicotine

If you are an avid coffee drinker as I was, then eliminating this beverage from your diet completely will be a challenge. Caffeine is a drug. I am not telling you to give up coffee for good.

That is up to you, although I do believe you would be better off if you did. But I do suggest that you keep its consumption to a bare minimum. I was a coffee fanatic. Yet, once I got used to drinking non-caffeinated tea, I felt better than ever and did not miss coffee at all.

If You Smoke

I was a pack-a-day smoker for 15 years and know how hard it is to quit. I don't have the space in this report to get into quitting methods, but I do have a resource that I believe will help. Visit Become an EX and follow the program indicated. When I made the decision, I stopped puffing immediately while doing a 40-day water fast. It was very hard for the first 7-to-10 days, but then I was free. I strongly urge you to make the decision to quit and use this report as the springboard to being smoke-free once and for all.

About Alcohol Consumption

While I certainly am not here to tell you not to drink, I do recommend that during this process you abstain from alcoholic beverages. Later on, once you have made some progress, you can decide for yourself which way you want to go.

Drinking an occasional glass of wine or beer is fine for most people, but your new fasting and detox lifestyle is best served by moderation and honesty.

If you find yourself drinking more than you should, then the time may come for you to consider quitting for good. That in itself can fill up pages and pages and is not in the scope of what we are working on here. If you think you may have a drinking problem, a simple Google search will rapidly avail you of some positive resources.

Going Past the Hunger Barrier

You have some experience with fasting, so you are probably not a stranger to hunger pangs and other symptoms. However, once the fast is over and you begin the standard diet, you will find yourself face-to-face with a new series of challenges. Keep in mind:

You are stepping into uncharted waters and beginning a deep physical, mental and emotional transformation.

Many people ask me: What can I expect to go through while on this standard diet?

You will likely feel hungry most of the time

You will likely get angry and frustrated because you can't eat more

You may find yourself mentally planning a binge

You will likely be moody

You will likely become impatient because 'this isn't happening fast enough'

You may find yourself rationalizing 'why you can't do this right now.'

You'll likely find plausible arguments to justify giving up and eating whatever you want

You will likely get sick of cooking

You will crave the very foods you have eliminated from your diet

You may forget why you are doing this in the first place (to achieve permanent weight loss and health)

You may convince yourself that you would rather regain all of the weight and try later than to continue. "I just want to eat what I want, when I want it!"

You may feel sad and want to cry

You may dream about food

Believe it or not, this is all perfectly normal and WILL pass; the hunger will lessen over time as you become increasingly used to eating clean, healthy foods. Furthermore, you will be developing crucial mental and physical tools that will help you to master food and hunger, instead of the other way around. Positive change is never easy, especially when we confront negative patterns that have been with us for years. One thing is certain:

Change may be difficult, but it is <u>ALWAYS</u> worthwhile.

When you make it to the other side and experience that amazing sense of freedom and wellbeing, the sacrifices that you endured along the way will seem small and insignificant.

Right now, make a commitment with yourself that, no matter what, you are going to stick it out and complete this 30-day program.

What About After Day 30?

After you complete the 30 days re-feeding process, it will be important for you to put together a structured eating program that you can follow in perpetuity, or at the very least for nine months. To this end, I wrote <u>The Permanent Weight Loss Diet</u>. In it, I give you a detailed presentation of the long-term diet that has helped me to keep the weight off for more than ten years. I encourage you to read it and incorporate it as part of your long-term maintenance phase.

Here, however, are some tips that can help you once you've completed the 30 days:

Stay away from sugar as much as you possibly can. Stick with the corn tortillas as a bread substitute. If you are a big breakfast fan as I am, then go ahead and eat no more than two eggs (*no more than three eggs weekly*) and two slices of lean ham or turkey, but **DO NOT** eat any bacon or sausage! Butter is forbidden. Use the "*no-stick*" nonfat Spam spray for cooking.

Packaged turkey and ham must be rinsed in water to remove excess salt before consumption.

Please do not eat any of it straight out of the package. If you are able, I suggest you purchase deli ham and turkey and avoid the pre-packaged ones. If you eat hash browns or breakfast potatoes, **DO NOT** fry them! I actually cook mine in water with a pinch of salt and allow the heat to brown them. It may not be as tasty as frying them, but you'll get used to it. You can have grits, but it should not exceed one cup, and no more than twice per week.

Cheese should be avoided, but if you must, then have ONE slice per day, preferably of the lowest fat type that you can find. Cheese can take a whole report in itself. I strongly encourage you to not eat cheese as it often prolongs cravings. Do not eat more than one slice of any type of cheese per day. I know that I said this before, but here it is again: **Stay away from refined sugar**. Stick with apples, oranges, strawberries and cantaloupe. Eat them whole or juice them. Do not overindulge, however, on heavier fruits like bananas and honeydew. Limit avocadoes as they are high on fat. If you drink orange juice for breakfast, do not let it exceed one cup. Most supermarket brand orange juices have way too much sugar. The same goes for apple, cranberry and grape juice. Only one cup of **ONE** of them, <u>ONCE</u> a day!

After you eat breakfast, do not eat anything else for at least four hours. If you become hungry and the cravings/hunger pains start to strike – *as they almost always do* – then your secret weapon is to drink a large glass of water quickly. If that does not work, drink another glass and **tell your stomach to shut up.**

In between meals, you can drink seltzer water with a pinch of lime. Some brands of seltzer already come with lime. But do not overdo it with the seltzer because, for some people, this may irritate the stomach. If your tummy is ok with seltzer, then you can drink more of it. Drink small amounts for several days until you are able to gauge how your stomach reacts.

For lunch & dinner, follow the same guideline of no sugar, butter or bread. Make sure that – *at least for dinner* – you eat a healthy salad. You must eat at least one salad per day. I also strongly encourage you to eat steamed vegetables with either lunch or dinner. If you want to eat steak, go ahead and do so – but make sure you cut out all of the fat and cook it to at least medium. The steak should not exceed 8 oz.

Eat more fish. Tilapia is my personal favorite, but go ahead and experiment. If you're a big meat eater, this may seem like a tall order. But believe me, the body will react. Eventually you will find yourself gravitating to fish or chicken over meat. I used to eat meat almost every day, but now I find that it gives me an uncomfortable sense of fullness. I read in a medical journal some years ago that most adult *"carnivores"* have large chunks of *"undigested meat"* in their bowels, just sitting there rotting. That information definitely served to motivate me.

A span of at least six hours should pass between lunch and dinner. Use the water, seltzer, green tea techniques outlined above to deal with hunger pains and cravings. Remember, the cravings and hunger pains will lessen over time. **That is the best news I can give you!** They do lessen and eventually, in most cases, vanish altogether! After dinner, you may find hunger creeping back in before you go to bed. Have a cup of no-fat yogurt mixed with fruits as outlined above for the breakfast portion. Have a couple of glasses of water after that. Seltzer with lime is fine. I do not recommend you drink green tea at night because it may keep you awake since it does have some caffeine.

Personally, I would suggest you cut out the caffeine altogether and purchase the non-caffeinated green tea instead. So this is basically how I manage my eating from day to day. In a few months I will have gone **TEN** years without binging or gaining any weight back. And the same can happen for you; IF you have the courage to take action.

The Road Ahead

This content has the potential to change the course of your life. If followed closely, it can literally break the chains of poor eating, constant weight gain and toxicity. Many people I share this system with immediately see drastic results physically and emotionally. Their overall perspective on life changes and they feel renewed. But please: Remember that this must be done **ONE DAY AT A TIME.**

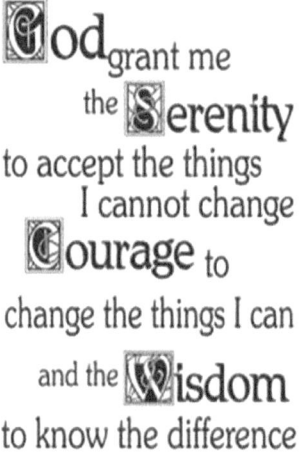

God grant me
the Serenity
to accept the things
I cannot change
Courage to
change the things I can
and the Wisdom
to know the difference

The big breakthrough comes by doing the right thing each day over a period of time. Stop thinking about how much "*time*" you have left to go; and just focus on what you have to do **NOW**. Saying the **SERENITY PRAYER** is by far my favorite way to bring myself back to center when I become overwhelmed. If you work at maintaining this simple perspective, staying on a clean diet will be **MUCH** easier. Eventually, it will become second nature.

You have all of the tools that you need to do it. All you need is a genuine desire, and the willingness to take action. If you can muster that, then great things will happen! Yes, it can get tough. But it is very much worth it. What is the alternative? To return to obesity, poor eating and eventual illness? NO! We must push forward with faith and perseverance. And so, the road is now before you... what will your choice be?

The Mental Battle

In closing, I want to share with you an excerpt of a correspondence I had recently with one of my coaching clients. I think the context will help to solidify your understanding of the task at hand.

"In our sessions, we have covered a **LOT** of ground related to the mind, related to your tendency to overeat, related to the rebellious part inside of us that despises structure and '*wants to do what it wants to do.*' We have talked about learning to identify the thoughts, impulses and feelings that want to lead you astray. We've talked about the importance of resisting these urges, thoughts and feelings, understanding that giving in to them will only set you back and take you away from your goals. **Is that not exactly what happens when you give in?** The eating structure that we put together is very personal to you and it is perfect. I am certain that it works.

The problem is that you continue to listen to those voices, agree with them and then **DO** what they suggest like: "*eat that cheese now, you want it, you need it, you deserve it!*" Whatever is causing you to stray from the eating plan is strictly in the mind. <u>YOU</u> getting angry because you feel deprived, allowing laziness to control you because you don't want to cook, rationalizing that you've done enough and that now you *'should be able to eat whatever you want, whenever you want.'* **THAT** is the crux of the problem. I faced it myself, so I know what I'm talking about.

The **VICTORY** that you want will come <u>ONLY</u> when you stop fighting the process, when you embrace the eating plan and learn to see it as your doorway to freedom. As long as you keep fighting, wanting to do this **YOUR** way, it will never work. The war is over. Put down your weapons. Move over to the winning side (*your eating plan and healthy lifestyle*). You must place your entire focus on getting good at following the eating plan and resisting the thoughts, urges and feelings that invite you to stray. That's the key to breakthrough, transformation and permanent weight loss.

Choose to stick to the eating plan and **RESIST, RESIST, RESIST** everything that leads you away from your objective. You must come to realize that those old thoughts, impulses and urges are, in essence, your enemy. Would you be willing to agree and do what is suggested by someone you know is your enemy? I don't think so. I think that, if you knew someone was your enemy, you would promptly reject anything this person offered. So I ask you, if those old thoughts, impulses and urges are your enemy, why do you continue to agree with them and follow their suggestions?

Why do you betray yourself by agreeing and acting on these voices? It is betrayal, is it not? You know that those voices, urges, thoughts and feelings only wish to lead you to overeat which, in turn, will move you away from your goal. You **KNOW** that these urges, voices, thoughts and feelings mean you no good, do you not? Of course you do! **Then why do you continue to go with them?** You must resist! Even if it feels like your arm will fall off if you don't eat that piece of cheese, or whatever... you **<u>MUST</u>** get mad and **RESIST**! The time has come for you to finally, once and for all, disconnect and destroy all of those negative voices, thoughts and impulses that come from old (*and counterproductive*) habits.

Stop walking through the old path! Refuse to walk through it. Instead, walk through the new path which is your eating plan and all of the great things that it will bring to your life – **IF** you stick to it. Make that new path clearer before you by using it constantly. Let the old path grow weeds and close down from lack of use.

The enemy is your stubborn insistence on listening to, agreeing with and acting on what the old habits tell you.

<u>THAT</u> is what is causing you to slip off the wagon and regain weight. But, **TODAY**, you can turn it around by saying **ENOUGH IS ENOUGH!** I will not be a puppet to the desires of my mind, body and belly! I am going to be free! I follow my eating plan with gladness because it is leading me to victory. It is leading me to triumph over the old habits, and – *one day* – I will be completely free of the urge to overeat. And those urges will never <u>EVER</u> be able to control me again.

You have made a <u>LOT</u> of progress and you have seen evident results. But to keep the progress and the results requires a bit of sacrifice. Sacrifice by refusing to give in to the old voices and – instead – affirming the new lifestyle by holding steady to your eating plan. **Regardless of how you feel or what the mind may say – stick to the eating plan.** You feel angry, lazy and deprived? Stick to the eating plan! You feel that you deserve to splurge? Reject it and stick to the eating plan! I want you to KILL those old habits... reject their invitations and revoke their power over you; refuse to do what they ask. It is the internal conversation with the old habits which has caused you to slip. You <u>MUST</u> move your focus away from the old habits and start reinforcing the new ones. How? By reinforcing your healthy eating plan and understanding that sticking to it is your doorway to freedom. Understand, in your heart of hearts, that the old habits represent an internal enemy that, if heeded, will ALWAYS lead you back to bondage – away from all of your cherished goals. I am placing the solution in front of you and explaining how it works and what you must do to seize it. But you must take that plunge. You must stop agreeing with your enemies, agreeing with those who wish to hold you back. It is time for you to get good at this, to master it! Do that, and the old habits will diminish and become a minor irritation. You will have created a new, healthy lifestyle filled with liberty, courage, commitment, sacrifice ... freedom!"

Until next time, God Bless and Godspeed!

ROBERT DAVE JOHNSTON

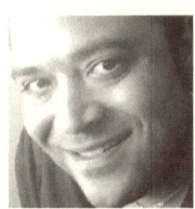

Grab The Entire Collection!

How to Lose Weight Fast, Keep it Off & Renew the Mind, Body & Spirit through Fasting, Smart Eating & Practical Spirituality

Volume 1: The 'Permanent Weight Loss' Diet

Volume 2: The Intermittent Fasting Weight Loss Formula

Volume 3: How to Lose 30 Pounds (Or More) In 30 Days With Juice Fasting

Volume 4: Burn the Blubber; How to Lose Belly Fat Fast, and For Good!

Volume 5: Lose the Emotional Baggage: Transform Your Mind & Spirit With Fasting

Volume 6: How to Break a Fast and Keep the Weight Off

Volume 7: How to Lose 40 Pounds (Or More) in 30 Days with Water Fasting

Also by Robert Dave Johnston:

Binge Free – Triumph Over Binge Eating, Confessions of a Former Food Addict, Volume 1

How to Lose weight & Keep it Off by Transforming the Mind & Behaviors

Volume 1: How to Lose Weight & Keep it Off By Reprogramming the Subconscious Mind

Volume 2: Mental Strategies to Defeat Diet Hunger and Junk Food Cravings

Volume 3:The Cravings Ninja Assassin

Volume 4: How to Cheat On Your Diet (And Get Away With It)

Volume 5: Compilation: SAVE BIG: Get All 5 For the Price of 3

Detoxify Your Body, Lose Weight, Get Healthy & Transform Your Life

Volume 1: The 10-Day 'At-Home' Colon Cleansing Formula

Volume 2: Bug Off! A 30-Day Parasite, Liver, Kidney Detox & Weight Loss Plan

Volume 3: Lose 30 Pounds (Or More) in 30 Days with Intermittent Fasting & Coffee Enemas

Volume 4: Compilation: Get All 3 for the Price of 2

Don't forget to check the articles and growing health community at: FitnessThroughFasting.com

Rob's first work of horror/fiction has just been released.
King of Pain – A Journey to Hell & Back Through the Mind's Eye Volume 1 – The Descent

www.ingramcontent.com/pod-product-compliance
Lightning Source LLC
Chambersburg PA
CBHW050425290526
45786CB00003B/1400